Ketogenic Diet book for beginners

Stella Parker

Table of Content

Introduction

I would like you to know first of how much I appreciate your gesture of purchasing and downloading this book.

This book has been very carefully designed to let you know everything there is to know about a Ketogenic Diet, even if you are an absolute beginner!

Throughout the whole book, I will be discussing the core concepts of Ketogenic Diet while introducing you to some interesting recipes for you to start experimenting on your own!

You should keep in mind though that once you have started up a Ketogenic Diet regime, you should always try to maintain it for as long as possible. Falling out from the diet might result in adverse effects. However, if you can follow through, then greatness awaits!

Welcome, to the world of Ketogenic Diet!

Chapter 1: The Burning Question, Does The Keto Diet Work?

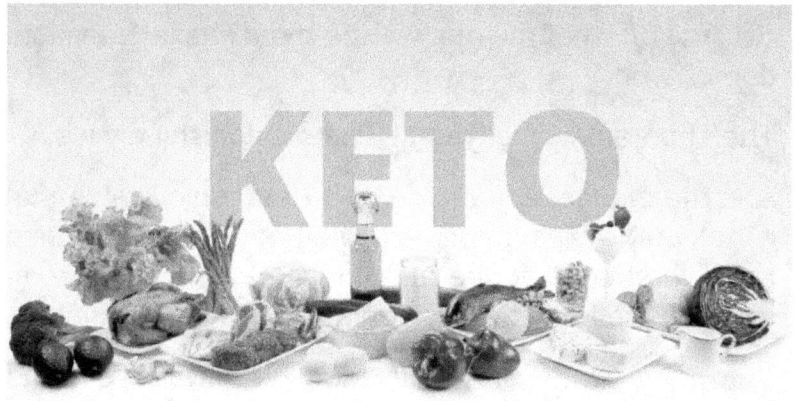

All of a sudden in our modern age, there has been a massive explosion that is catapulting the concept of Ketogenic Diet to the mouth of millions out there!

Even for individuals who are not entirely aware of what a "Ketogenic Diet" truly is, they are jumping on the hype wagon and are rushing towards doing thorough research and figuring out what the mysterious Ketogenic Diet is.

I am pretty sure that you are here for the same reason as well! You probably have heard of the Ketogenic Diet from a friend or family member, and you are now looking to dive into this world to trim down that excess body fat of yours, right?

Well, you've come to the right place!

But instead of drowning you in a sea of information, I am going to break down the whole concept into individual chunks for you to quickly absorb.

So, first off...Let me answer the most crucial question: does it work?

The short answer is, yes! It works astonishingly well!

And the biggest advantage of a Ketogenic Diet is that it not only helps to trim down body fat, but it also helps the body acquire an enhanced immune system, allowing the body to stay healthy for days to come!

But good word of mouth doesn't always cut the dough, right? Sometimes you need concrete evidence to believe something, right?

But you have probably all of these before, right? Let me hold your hand and walk you through a recent study which takes the concept of Ketogenic Diet for a spin.

A team of eight different and well-known experts were hired to undertake an extensive study to test the efficacy of the Atkins Diet (A very close cousin to the Ketogenic Diet) over a span of 12 months, by comparing it to the Zone, Ornish, and LEARN diets.

An average age of 41 years was measured of the sample, following a BMI of 32 with body fat which clocked at a percentage of 40%

After establishing these basal standards, the scientists divide the whole sample into four different groups based on the type of diet they were exposed to.

Once the measuring standards were signified, the experiment was then established The 311 individuals into four different groups for the study.

- Group-1 comprised of 76 people and were exposed to Ornish Diet with 10% lowered down calorie count.
- Group 2 had 79 participants, and they were asked to go through a LEARN Diet which comprised of the same 10% fewer calories, but this time it came from the saturated fats, while 55-60% of the calorie came from the carbohydrates.
- Group 3 comprising of 79 people was exposed to something called the "Zone Diet" which consisting of roughly 30%, 40% and 30% distribution of calories coming from protein, carbohydrate and fats respectively.
- The last group had 77 individuals, and they were treated to an Atkins Diet.

So, you can see that the test was incredibly elaborate and thoroughly thought out. If you want to skip out on all of the complicated explanations, then just have a look at the graph below!

With that being said, you can now clearly understand how large and elaborate the test was. However, I don't want to bore you with a complicated explanation! Instead, have a look at the graph below which would easily give you the result of the experiment!

Just at a glance, you would immediately notice that Atkins Diet had a significant effectiveness when it came to lowering down the weight.

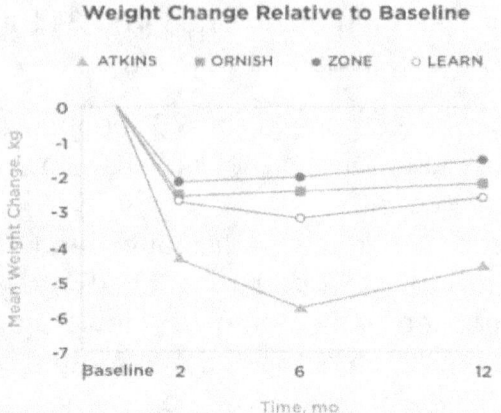

Credit: Taken from www.ruled.me

The same is seen in the bar chart below.

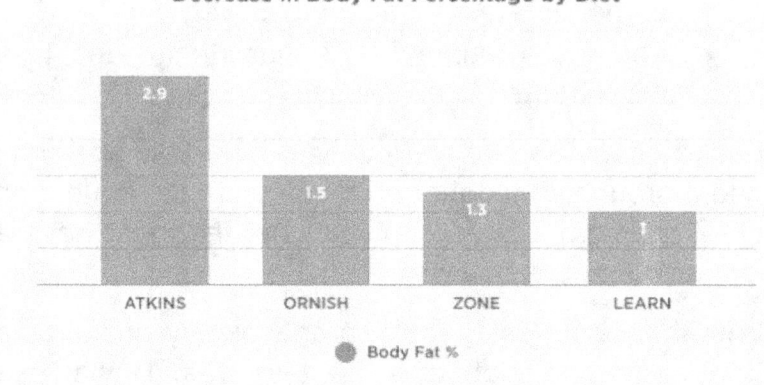

Credit: Taken from www.ruled.me

But that's not the only thing the researchers got from the experiment! The body fat percentage of the individuals also had very positive results regarding Atkins in comparison to the other diets.

The recorded rate decrease from the Atkins diet was at an astounding 2.9% while the others had a decline of around 1.5%, 1.3% and 1% in the Ornish, Zone, and LEARN group respectively. Which even further supports the theory of the effectiveness of a low carb diet.

The conclusion then? Atkins Diet and in turn Ketogenic Diet can help to trim down the body fat in no time! And make you healthier as well!

Chapter 2: Getting The Concept Of Body Weight

In this chapter, though, I am going to ask you take a step backward before moving forth!

Why do you ask? Because before being able to understand the how Ketogenic Diet works fully, it is essential that you know a little bit about how your body deals with weight and fat.

Everyone pretty much these days is always discussing amongst their peers and researching around the web on how to lose their body weight and turn into the next hot superstar!

But have you ever wondered, when we are talking about "Weight," what exactly are we referring to?

Well, in Layman's term we are talking about the mass of our body. The bulk mass that comes from the amount of water, bones, body fat and muscle in our body.

Everything that makes up the whole skeletal infrastructure comprises our mass.

Following that definition, when a person is referred to as being either "Fat" or even "Obese," they are being said that they have a significant amount of body fat or "mass" that is hampering their overall body physique and health.

Professionals such as Doctors or Nurses, though, often follow something which is called the BMI or Body Mass Index.

Curious to know what BMI is? Well, again in Layman's term, BMI is a method of measurement which is done by comparing the height and weight of an individual. The BMI value is then later on use using the formula and the chart below to get an idea of a person's physique.

$$\text{Body Mass Index} = \frac{\text{Weight (in kg)}}{\text{Height}^2 \text{ (in m)}}$$

The standards you see in the graph were set by an extensive research done by the World Health Organization, so they are extremely accurate. So, imagine that you have a body index of 25-30, it would make you overweight. Alternatively, if you have an index of 30+, you would be obese.

Sadly, though, at the time of writing, the level of people suffering from obesity and a high body fat percentage was at an all-time high. In fact, in 2014 it was estimated that almost 600 million adults were suffering from obesity while 42 million of the total obese population were children under five! Thank you excellent fast foods!

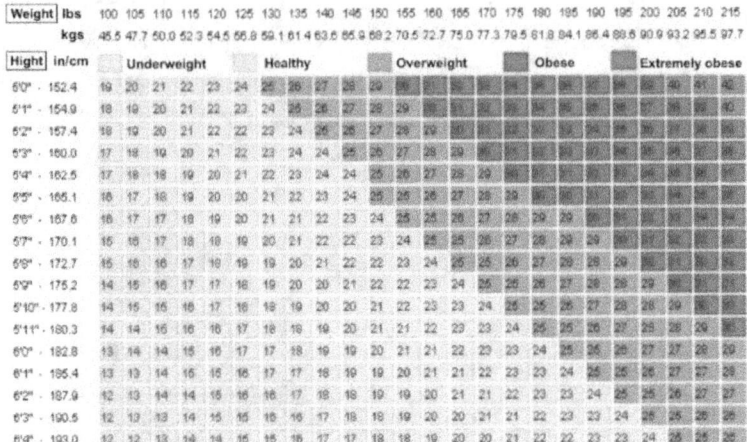

Credit: Taken from Healthy and Natural World

From the chart above, you will easily be able to assess if you are under the category of being underweight, healthy, overweight or even being obese.

Chapter 3: So, What Is Ketogenic Diet?

Now that you know a bit about your body weight let me walk you through the Ketogenic Diet now.

The Ketogenic Diet

The general definition of the word "Keto" is derived from a bodily metabolic process known as "Ketosis." This process is what allows to body to lose weight so fast while under a Ketogenic Diet.

In the simplest and Layman's terms, the definition of the word "Keto" is derived from a process known as Ketosis.

What is Ketosis you say? Well, it is the process through which the body releases a chemical called Ketones which significantly helps to lower down the level of fats in our body.

I will tell you how that works in just a bit.

But, let's get back to Ketogenic Diet first.

So, the primary aim of a Ketogenic Diet is to basically down your carbohydrate input to a very basal and minimal level, while at the same time doubling on your fat intake.

And this is precisely why Ketogenic Diet has also been known as a High-Fat-Low-carb Diet all around the world.

Thanks to that, Ketogenic Diet is also called "High-Fat-Low-Carb Diet" amongst people of different niche.

However, before fully explaining how a Ketogenic Diet works you need to learn to appreciate how the body controls its Glucose and Insulin levels.

To make things clear and easy, whenever our body is taking up a significant amount of Carbohydrate, the production or glucose and insulin start to rise as well.

One thing you should know, though, that Glucose is a pretty flexible convertible molecule, which the body uses whenever energy is required.

Alternatively, Insulin works as a means of countermeasure if the level of glucose in the bloodstream goes beyond normal levels. If the degree of glucose in the blood is low, insulin levels lower down. On the other hand, if the glucose level rises, insulin helps to lower it down.

You might be wondering now, what does all of these have to do with losing your weight right?

Well, whenever your body is in a constant supply of glucose, it starts to break it down rather than fat to get the energy! So, burning down Fat is entirely avoided here.

Even if you end up running all day and are in need of an energy boost, the fat just stays there in your body instead as the glucose is being burned for the energy, causing the fat to keep accumulating.

As long as you are on a high carbohydrate diet, the fat levels won't come down because the body is always breaking down Carbohydrates.

And this is where Ketogenic Diet kicks in!

Whenever your body is derived from a good supply of carbohydrate, it throws the body into a state of "Ketosis" where it will release the aforementioned chemicals called "Ketones."

Ketones then greatly help to encourage the burning down of fat from our body.

And Since fat is usually present in abundance in our body, the body always feels energetic to the core.

Advantages of Ketogenic Diet

So, about I let you know a bit about the different advantages and benefits of going into a Ketogenic Diet!

✓ A good Keto diet will help you to lower the levels of bad cholesterol so to prevent arterial blocks from occurring
✓ Energy taken from burning body fat will always keep you energetic since body fat is present in abundance in our body

✓ The levels of LDL will decrease which will make the body less prone to suffer from Type-2 Diabetes
✓ You won't always feel hungry
✓ Ketosis helps to improve skin condition and prevent acnes or skin inflammation from taking place.

But what about the other benefits of Ketogenic Diet, other than trimming down your weight you ask?

- A Ketogenic diet directly helps to increase the level of fat burnt throughout the whole day through exercise and daily activities
- A Keto Diet will cause the body to consume a significant amount of protein, consequently promoting the weight loss of the body.
- When the body is restricted from consuming Carbohydrates, the calorie intake will also lower down further contributing to weight loss.
- A process called Gluconeogenesis will kick in as well which will cause the body to burn even more fat.
- Speaking of burning fat, A Ketogenic diet will also help you to Suppress your Appetite, so you won't have to go out and eat now and then and bulk up, even more, fat.

Chapter 4: All You Need To Know About Ketosis

The signs and symptoms of Ketosis

I have already explained to you "What Ketosis" is right? But how are you going to understand that you have entered into a state of Ketosis anyways? It's not as hard as you might think actually! Just check for the following signs and symptoms.

- Your mouth will feel dry, and you feel have increased thirst
- The number of washroom visits will increase as you might need to urinate more often.
- Your breath will have a slight "Fruity" smell to it that will resemble that of a nail polish
- Aside from those three, you will obviously get the sensation mentioned above of having a low hunger level and increased bodily energy.

Entering the optimal levels of Ketosis

By now you should have a bright idea that Ketogenic Diet primarily starts working when you have entered into a state of Ketosis right?

While you certainly can enter Ketosis by just going through some simple steps, the following will not only enhance the effectiveness of Ketosis but also allow your body to sustain and keep itself in a Ketosis state for a prolonged period.

- Keep your daily carbohydrate intake below 20 carbs
- Keep your protein levels at around 70g per day
- Don't starve! Swallow adequate level of fat. Remember that the body is going to need fat to burn fat.
- Try to avoid snack times and stick to your breakfast, lunch and dinner meals with nothing in between.

The effects of Keto on your body

Aside from your fat levels, a Ketogenic Diet will bring some different changes to the overall homeostatic functions of your body.

The body has to start generating enough enzymes to deal with the Keto Meals.

This change requires the body to go through a broad alteration process which sometimes results from a number of minor side effects.

During the very early stages of starting a Ketogenic Diet, you might be experiencing some of the following symptoms alongside just a general feeling of lethargy.

- Dizziness
- Aggravation
- Headaches
- Keto-Flu
- Mental Fogginess

Chapter 5: Tips for your Keto Diet and Mistakes to avoid!

Now you are nearly ready to start off your journey! But below are a few quick tips which will help you to Kickstart your Keto diet quest effortlessly.

- Buy a counter to keep track of your carb intake.
- Toss out all of the high-carb produces from your kitchen.
- Pack up your pantry with only Keto suitable produces.
- Makeup and follow a strict meal plan
- Try to give up your old habits and pursue newer, healthier habits.
- Keep yourself packed up with enough water to make sure that you can replenish the flushed out electrolytes.

Once you have decided that you are going to jump into a Ketogenic Diet, one thing which you might find interesting to follow is a technique known as "Intermittent fasting."

This tells you that you should start a pre-phase of low carb diets before actually starting the diet itself, to allow your body to adjust and re-orient itself to the coming changes.

This fasting method is comprised of two phases. Namely the Building Phase (Time between first and last meal) and the cleaning phase (Time between last and first meal). Try to maintain a period of 12 hours between the cleansing phase and 8 hours between the building phases for a start. Then keep on growing from that.

- Make sure to keep your sodium intake in check to avoid future problems during your Ketogenic journey. Easy steps may include
  ✓ Drinking organic broth if possible
  ✓ Taking a just a pinch of pink salt with you consumed meals
  ✓ Adding about ¼ teaspoon of pink salt to 16 ounces of water consumed
  ✓ Adding vegetables such as kelp to your dishes
  ✓ Eating up vegetables such as cucumber or celery for a more natural approach to sodium replenishment
- It is essential to maintain a proper exercise routine to make sure that your body is in tip-top shape all throughout the regime.

With everything said and done, it should be mentioned now that there are some common mistakes which are made by new Keto enthusiasts.

- People often get confused regarding the fact of how many carbs they can consume per day. The very basic standard carb count is that you should keep your carb intake somewhere around 20-50g with a maximum intake of 100-150g at best.

- It is essential that you keep your protein intake in check. Too much protein will cause the body to start burning up protein instead of Fat! So, try to keep a balance.
- A grave mistake which people makes is that they sometimes try to lower down the Fat intake as well, thinking that it will double the effectiveness of a Ketogenic Diet. However, that is completely wrong, and you should never skip out on your fat intake.
- Make sure to go for as much water as you can. While you are on a Ketogenic Diet, the body will start to flush away electrolytes which will make you weak. To tackle this effect, it is essential to keep your body fully hydrated at all time and have a good amount of salt as well.

- Monday: Resistance training for upper body (20 minutes)
- Tuesday: Resistance training for Lower Body (20 minutes)
- Wednesday: Long walk of 30 minutes
- Thursday: Resistance training for upper body (20 minutes)
- Friday: Resistance training for Lower Body (20 minutes)
- Sat/Sun: Recreational time.

Chapter 6: Ingredients to go for and to avoid!

Fats

Go For

- Saturated Fat like coconut oil ghee
- Monosaturated Fat like olive, macadamia, almond oil
- Polyunsaturated Omega 3s as sardines
- Medium Chain Triglycerides such as fatty acid
- Lard
- Chicken Fat
- Duck Fat
- Goose Fat

Not Go For

- Refined Fats and Oil as sunflower, soybean, corn oil, etc.
- Trans Fat such as margarine

Protein

Go For

- Grass fed meat
- Harvested seafood and wild caught meat
- Free-range organic egg
- Beef

- Lamb
- Goat
- Venison
- Pastured Pork
- Poultry

Not Go For

- Factory packed animal foods and produced

Vegetable

Go For

- Leafy green vegetables
- Low carb vegetables
- Swiss chard
- Bok Choy
- Lettuce
- Chard
- Chives
- Endives
- Radicchio

Not Go For

- High starchy= high carb vegetables such as peas, potatoes, yucca, beans, legumes.

Dairy Products

Go For

- Dairy products such as yogurt, sour cream, cottage cheese, goat cheese

Not Go For

- Milk

Fruits

Go For

- In general, go for fruits that are on low carb and have more fat such as berries, avocados, etc.

Not Go For

- Try to avoid dried fruits that are high in sugar content

Drinks

Go For

- Water
- Black Coffee
- Unsweetened and Herbal Teas
- Nut Milks
- Light Beet
- Wine

Not Go For

- Drinks such as Pepsi or Coke
- High Fructose Syrup
- Nectar
- Honey
- Sodas

Sweets

Go For

- Stevia
- Xylitol
- Erythritol
- Inulin
- Monk Fruit Powder
- Cocoa Dark Chocolate

Not Go For

- Milk

Chapter 7: A Brief Look Into The Recipes

Shredded Salsa Chicken

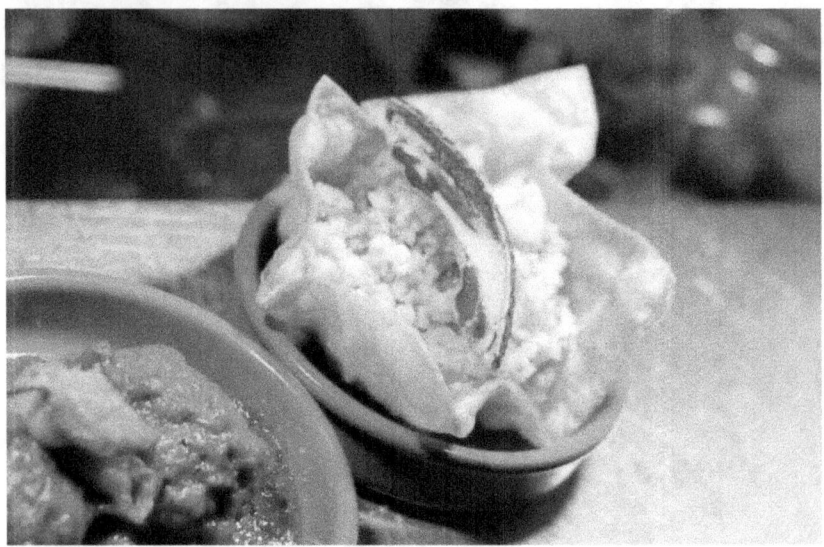

Time to prepare and cook

The recipe will take about 10 minutes to prepare and 15 minutes to cook

Ingredients

- 1 pound of chicken breast
- 1 and a ½ cup of salsa
- ½ a teaspoon of salt
- ¼ a teaspoon of black pepper
- ½ a teaspoon of onion powder
- ½ a teaspoon of garlic powder
- Cumin or paprika if needed

- Seeded jalapenos as required

Process

1. The first step of this dish is to toss in all of the ingredients into your Instant Pot and keep stirring it nicely
2. Close down the lid and select the poultry setting and let it cook for about 15 minutes at high pressure
3. Once done, let the pressure release quickly and remove the lid
4. Shred up the chicken with forks and serve with fresh cilantro and avocado slices

Nutrition

- Calories: 148
- Fat: 7.1g
- Carbohydrates: 17.2g
- Protein: 2.6g

Tomato-Poached Eggs

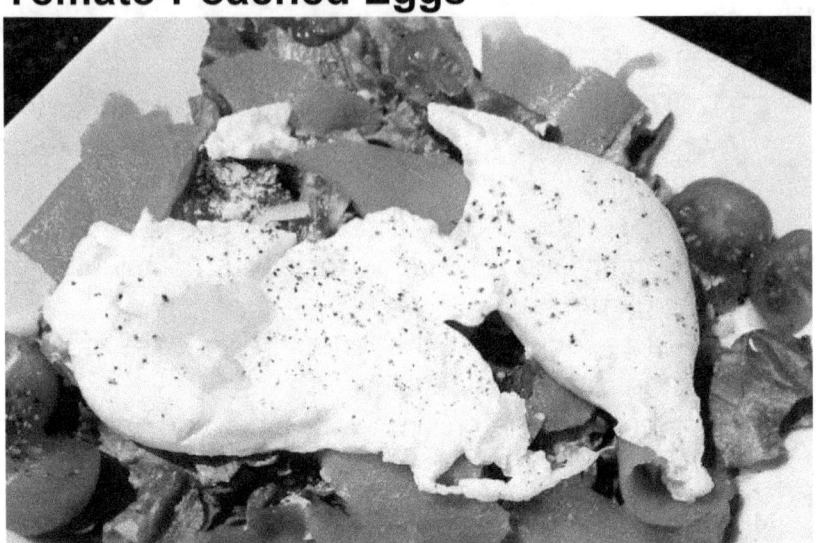

Time to prepare and cook

The recipe will take about 5 minutes to prepare and 5 minutes to cook.

Ingredients

- 5 large sized eggs
- 5 large sized tomatoes
- 3 tablespoon of melted butter
- ½ a teaspoon of pepper

Process

1. The first step here is to place about one cup of water in your inner pot
2. Hollow out your tomatoes by digging out the middle part of the vegetable
3. Take an egg and break it on each tomato and place those tomatoes on a dish

4. Place that dish on your Instant pot
5. Choose the pressure cooking mode and let it cook at low pressure for 5 minutes
6. Gently remove the eggs and top them off with pepper and butter
7. Gently serve it with turkey, beef slice or ham as you required

Nutrition

- Calories: 200
- Fat: 0g
- Carbohydrates: 0g
- Protein: 0g

Spicy Bacon Chicken

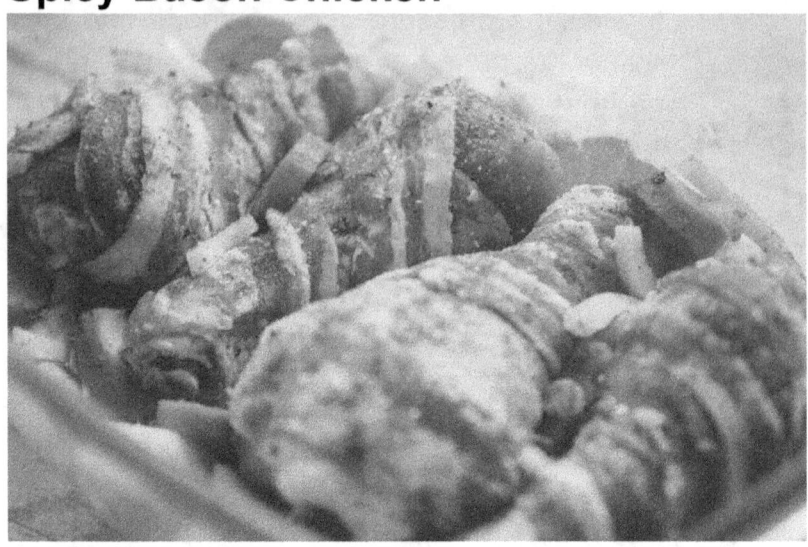

Time to prepare and cook

The recipe will take about 5 minutes to prepare and 25 minutes to cook.

Ingredients

- 2 pieces of chicken breast
- 1 cup of chicken broth
- 2 tablespoon of chili powder
- 2 jalapenos, chopped up
- 4 slices of fried and crispy bacon
- 1 cup of sour cream

Process

1. The first step here is to open up the lid of your instant pot and pour in the chicken broth in your inner pot

2. Toss in the jalapeno pepper and chili powder and keep mixing it gently
3. Toss in the chicken in your cooker and let it cook at high pressure for about 25 minutes
4. Once done, wait for 10 minutes and release the pressure naturally
5. Open the lid and pour in the sour cream and stir it in nicely
6. Take it out and gobble it up!

Nutrition

- Calories: 201
- Fat: 4g
- Carbohydrates: 8g
- Protein: 24g

Warm Chicken Salad

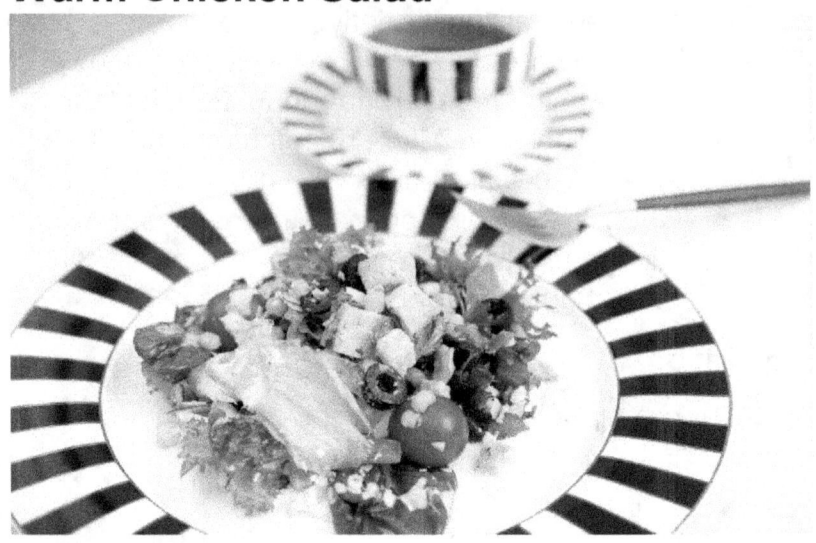

Time to prepare and cook

The recipe will take about 5 minutes to prepare and 30 minutes to cook.

Ingredients

- 1 whole piece of chicken
- 1 cup of water
- 1 cup of sour cream
- 1 teaspoon of garlic powder
- 1 teaspoon of black pepper
- 3 cup of baby spinach
- 3 diced up tomatoes
- 1 sliced up avocado

Process

1. The first step is to open up you're the lid of your instant pot and pour in water in your inner pot
2. Toss in your chicken
3. Set the instant pot on poultry mode and let it cook at high pressure for about 30 minutes
4. While that is being cooked, prepare your salad by taking a bowl and toss in the tomatoes, spinach, avocado and finely mix it
5. Toss in your sour cream alongside garlic powder, sprinkled with black pepper
6. By this time, the chicken should be ready. Open up your instant pot and bring it out, only to cut it finely
7. Once cut up, pour in your dressing and serve it warm over your prepared salad.

Nutrition

- Calories: 417
- Fat: 31g
- Carbohydrates: 2.55g
- Protein: 29g

Bone Braised Beef Short Ribs

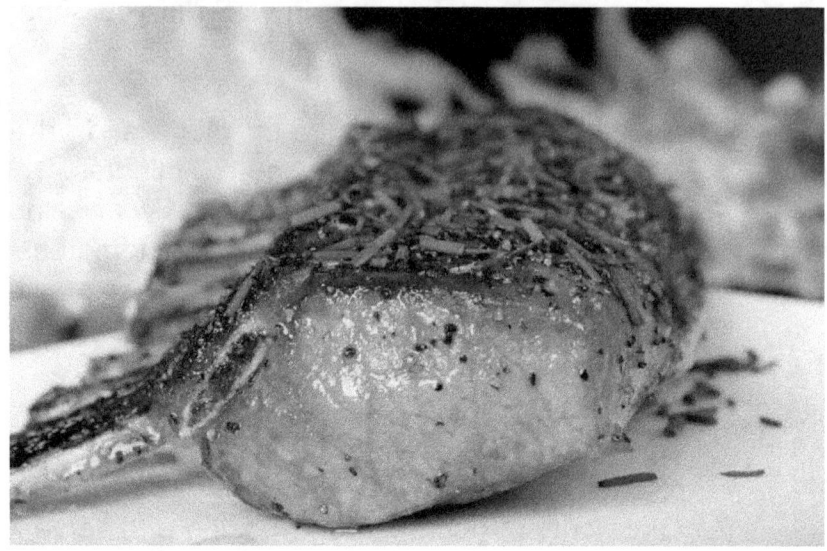

Time to prepare and cook

The recipe will take about 10 minutes to prepare and 35 minutes to cook.

Ingredients

- 4 pound of beef short ribs
- Generous amount of Kosher Salt
- 1 tablespoon of beef fat
- 1 quartered onion with its skin on
- 3 cloves of garlic
- Water

Process

1. Before beginning the cooking, you should first properly season the ribs with your preferred amount of salt

2. Take a skillet and heat up the beef oil over medium high. Toss in the ribs and gently cook them until browned
3. Once browned, toss in the garlic, onion and about 2 inches of water.
4. Once mixed, transfer the mixture to the instant pot and let it cook for about 35 minutes
5. Once the ribs complete, serve the dish with the dish on the bone
6. Alternatively, you can also pull the meat from the bones and braise the liquid and skim the fat. Store them in a jar and serve the ribs with the broth making sure to season them well.

Nutrition

- Calories: 550
- Fat: 39g
- Carbohydrates: 4g
- Protein: 14g

Corned Beef and Cabbage

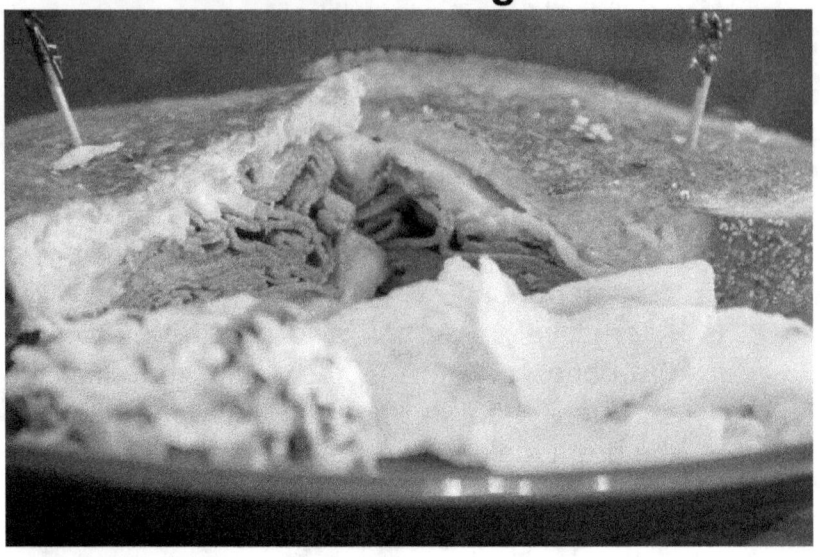

Time to prepare and cook

The recipe will take about 5 minutes to prepare and 2 hours to cook.

Ingredients

- 1 piece of corned beef brisket
- 4 cups of water
- 1 small sized peeled and quartered onion
- 3 cloves of peeled and smashed garlic clove
- 2 pieces of bay leaves
- 3 whole sized black peppercorns
- ½ a teaspoon of allspice berries
- 1 teaspoon of dried thyme
- 5 medium sized carrots
- 1 head of cabbage cut into wedges

Process

1. The first step is to toss in the corned beef, onion, water, garlic cloves, allspice, peppercorn, and thyme into your instant pot and close down the lid and set the timer to 90 minutes
2. Once the cooking is complete, turn off your device and allow the pressure to be excreted naturally.
3. Gently take out the meat and place them on a plate, only to cover them up with a tin foil and let it sit for just 15 minutes
4. Toss in the carrots and cabbage to the pot and lock up the lid, letting it cook for 10 minutes
5. Once the cooking is done, release the pressure quickly and take out the prepared vegetables and serve them alongside the corned beef.

Nutrition

- Calories: 478
- Fat: 25
- Carbohydrates: 3.8g
- Protein: 34.2g

Sweet Potato Gratin

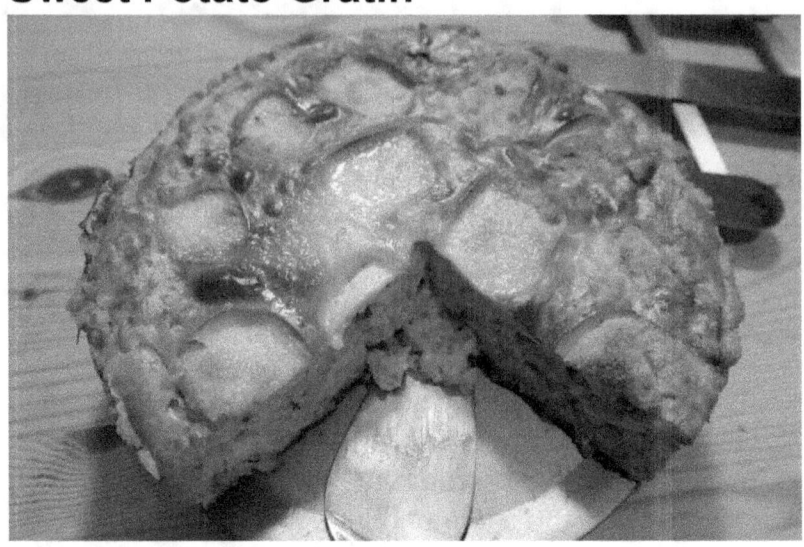

Time to prepare and cook

The recipe will take about 10 minutes to prepare and 9 minutes to cook

Ingredients

- 3 tablespoon of olive oil
- 3 cups of sliced up parsnips
- 3 cloves of chopped up garlic
- 2 cups of vegetable broth
- 1 tablespoon of black pepper
- 1 tablespoon of garlic powder
- 1 cup of cream cheese
- 2 cups of mozzarella cheese

Process

1. The first step here is to toss in all of your ingredients in the instant pot's inner pot except the cheddar cheese
2. Close up the lid and let it cook at high pressure for 5 minutes
3. Wait for about 10 minutes and let the pressure release naturally
4. Open up the lid and sprinkle mozzarella cheese all over
5. Set the instant pot to warm settings for about 5 minutes for the cheese to melt
6. Serve hot

Nutrition

- Calories: 201
- Fat: 10g
- Carbohydrates: 22g
- Protein: 6g

Veggie Stuffed Peppers

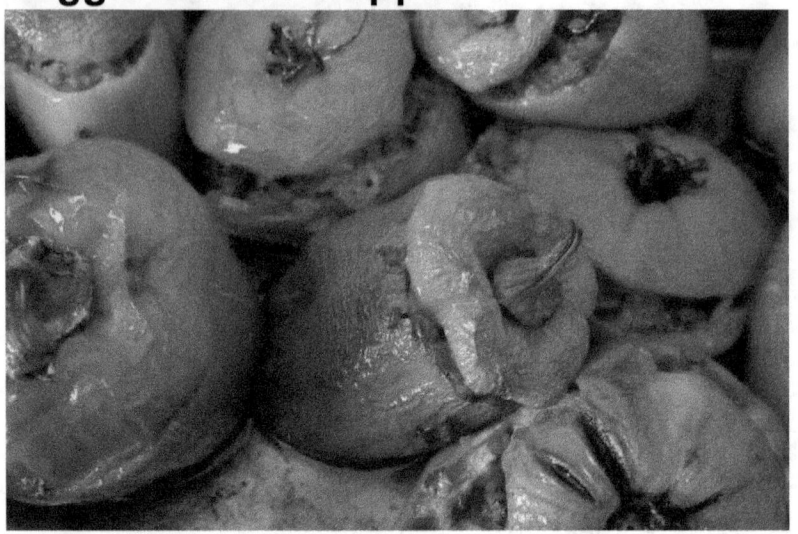

Time to prepare and cook

The recipe will take about 5 minutes to prepare and 16 minutes to cook with 8 serving

Ingredients

- 4 red bell peppers with their tops cut off
- 1 cup of white bean soaked overnight
- 1 cup of quinoa
- 1 cup of goat cheese
- 3 cups of vegetable broth
- 2 tablespoon of garlic powder

Process

1. Open up the lid of your pot and toss in the quinoa, beans, garlic powder and pour in the vegetable broth as well
2. Let it cook at high pressure for 8 minutes

3. Release the pressure naturally
4. Take your pepper and fill it up with bean and quinoa mixture
5. Wipe out your instant pot and place your filled in pepper in it
6. Change your instant pot mode to warm and keep it like that for 6 minutes.
7. Take it out and serve hot

Nutrition

- Calories: 313
- Fat: 24g
- Carbohydrates: 9g
- Protein: 15g

Zucchini and Cheese

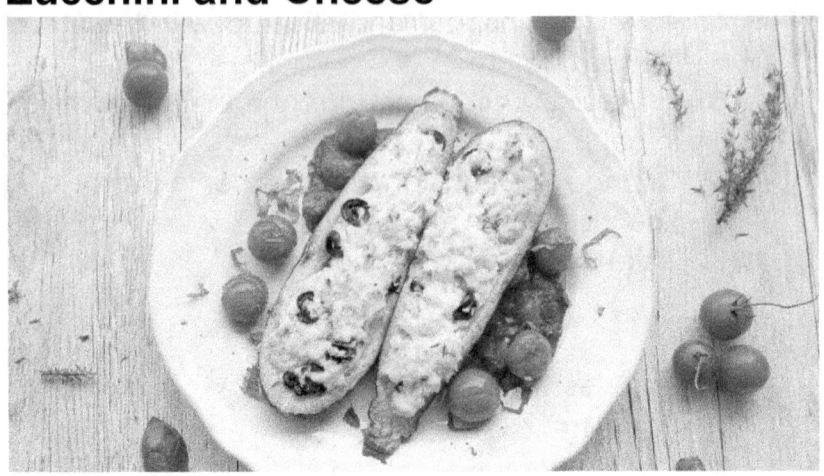

Time to prepare and cook

The recipe will take about 10 minutes to prepare and 4 minutes to cook with 4 serving.

Ingredients

- 3 tablespoon of olive oil
- 2 cup of zucchini
- 2 cups of spiralized carrots
- 3 chopped up garlic cloves
- 2 cups of vegetable broth
- 1 tablespoon of black pepper
- 1 tablespoon of garlic powder

Process

1. The first step is to toss in all of the ingredients in your instant pot
2. Cover up the lid and let it cook for about 4 minutes at high pressure

3. Once done, release the pressure naturally and serve it hot with some cheese sprinkled up

Nutrition

- Calories: 237
- Fat: 20g
- Carbohydrates: 7g
- Protein: 10g

Instant Pot Spicy Apple Cider

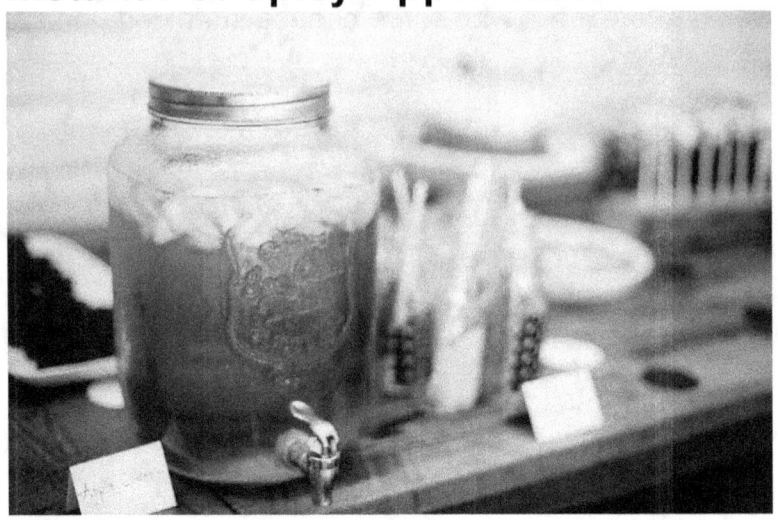

Time to prepare and cook

The recipe will take about 5 minutes to prepare and 6 minutes to cook with 4 servings

Ingredients

- 2 cups of moderately dry white wine
- ½ a cup of sugar
- ¼ teaspoon of grated nutmeg
- 1 piece of 4 inch cinnamon stick
- 8 whole cloves
- 4 pieces of large firm apples

Process

1. Take your wine, sugar, cinnamon stick, nutmeg, and cloves in your instant pot and sauté them until the sugar dissolves
2. Toss in your halved apples then and lock up the lid

3. Let it cook at high pressure for 6 minutes
4. Quick release the pressure
5. Unlock the pot and transfer the halves to a bowl
6. Bring the sauce in the pot to a medium heat and cook for 5 minutes, stirring it until the syrup is thickened
7. Discard the cinnamon sticks and cloves and pour the syrup over your apples

Nutrition

- Calories: 252
- Fat: 0g
- Carbohydrates: 30g
- Protein: 0g

Homemade Bolognese

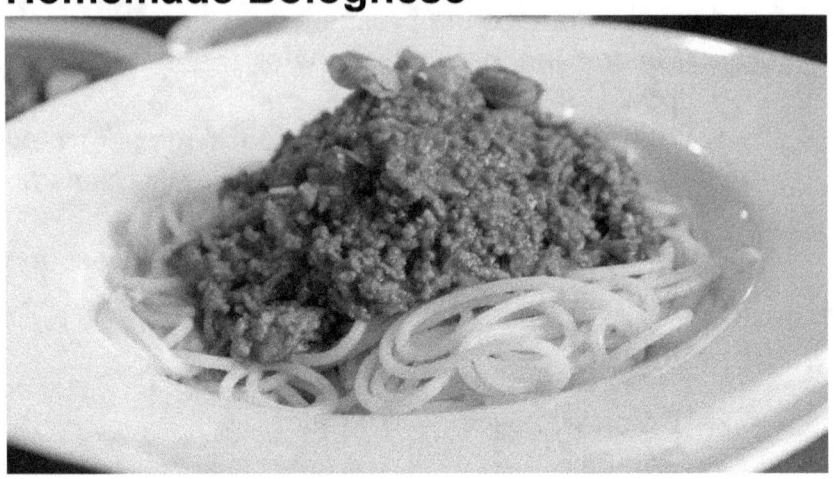

Time to prepare and cook

The recipe will take about 30 minutes to prepare and 10 minutes to cook with 8 servings

Ingredients

- 4 tablespoon of olive oil
- 1 and a ½ cup of finely chopped onion
- ¾ cup of finely chopped carrots
- ¾ cup of finely chopped celery
- 2 tablespoon of minced garlic
- ½ a pound of spicy Italian pork sausage
- ½ a pound of ground chunk
- 1 and a ½ teaspoon of kosher salt
- ¾ teaspoon of black pepper
- 2 teaspoon of ground fennel
- 1 teaspoon of Italian seasoning
- ½ a cup of red wine
- 1 can of crushed tomatoes
- 1 tablespoon of sugar

- 1 pound of cooked pasta
- Parmesan cheese

Process

1. This recipe is very straightforward and will only require you to set your pot to Saute Mode and pour in the oil
2. Toss in the carrots, onions, celery, garlic and Saute them nicely
3. Toss in the ground meat then followed by the seasoning and let it cook until the meat is perfectly browned up
4. Deglaze the pot with wine and cook for about 15 minutes
5. Stir while pouring tossing the tomatoes and sugar
6. Lock up the lid and let it cook at high pressure for 15 minutes
7. Once done, serve with spaghetti with sprinkles of parmesan cheese

Nutrition

- Calories: 237
- Fat: 14g
- Carbohydrates: 14g
- Protein: 16g

Sausage and Pepper

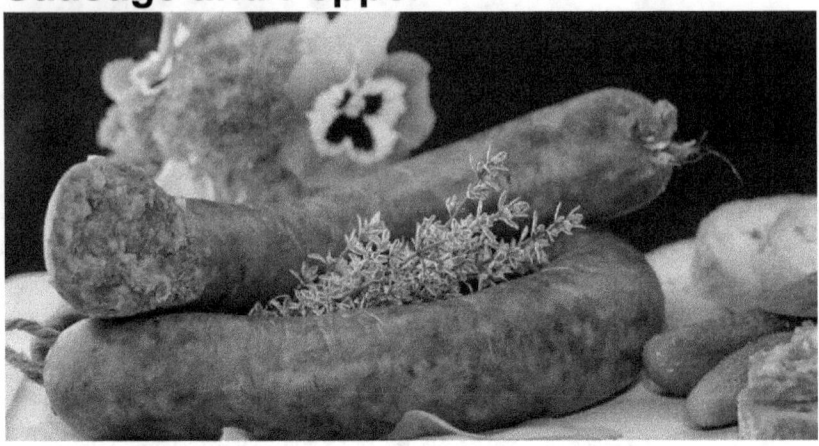

Time to prepare and cook

The recipe will take about 5 minutes to prepare and 10 minutes to cook with 8 servings

Ingredients

- 2 pound of Italian Sausage
- 2 sliced up bell peppers
- 2 chopped up Zucchini
- 1 chopped up onion
- 28 ounce of Italian stewed tomatoes
- 16 ounce of pasta sauce
- ½ a pound of dry penne pasta
- 1 and a ½ tablespoon of Italian seasoning
- Grated Parmesan cheese

Process

1. Start off the recipe by removing the sausage meat from their personal casing and tossing them to your instant pot.
2. Saute them until nicely browned up

3. Drain the fat from your cooker and toss in the garlic, peppers, and onions and let it cook for another 3 minutes
4. Stir in the remaining ingredients and pour just enough water to cover the ingredients up
5. Lock up the lid and let it cook at high pressure for 8 minutes
6. Naturally, release the pressure and open the lid
7. Transfer the mixture to your serving plate and serve with grated parmesan as garnish

Nutrition

- Calories: 288
- Fat: 21g
- Carbohydrates: 9g
- Protein: 14g

Maple Brown Rice

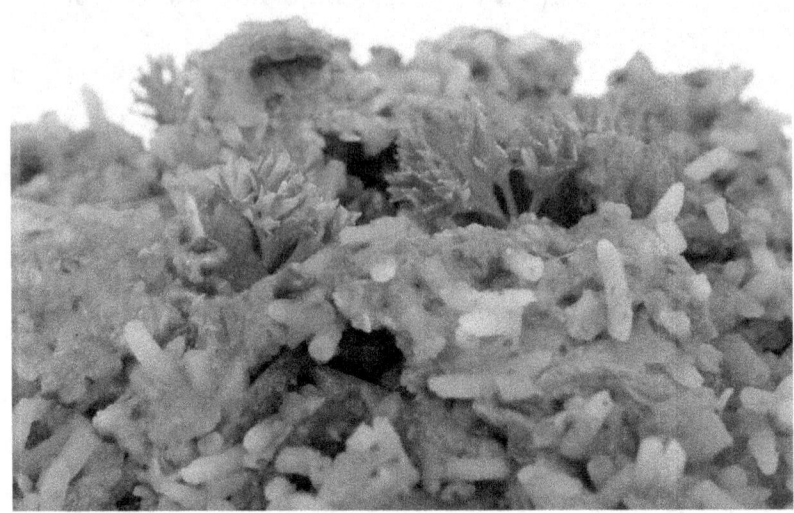

Time to prepare and cook

The recipe will take about 5 minutes to prepare and 10 minutes to cook with 4 servings

Ingredients

- 1 cup brown rice
- 1 and a ½ cup of water
- 2 tablespoon of maple syrup

Process

1. Open up the lid of your cooker and toss in the ingredients listed
2. Let it cook for 8 minutes at high pressure
3. Gently release the pressure naturally
4. Open it up bask in finely made Maple Brown Rice

Nutrition

- Calories: 226
- Fat: 0g
- Carbohydrates: 58g
- Protein: 0g

Conclusion

Before wrapping the book, I would like to take a moment here and tell you how much I appreciate you going through the whole book.

I really do hope that you enjoyed this book as much as I enjoyed writing it. Keep in mind that with this book you just scratched the tip of the iceberg! Keep exploring.

Be prepared and may you stay safe and healthy!

God Bless!

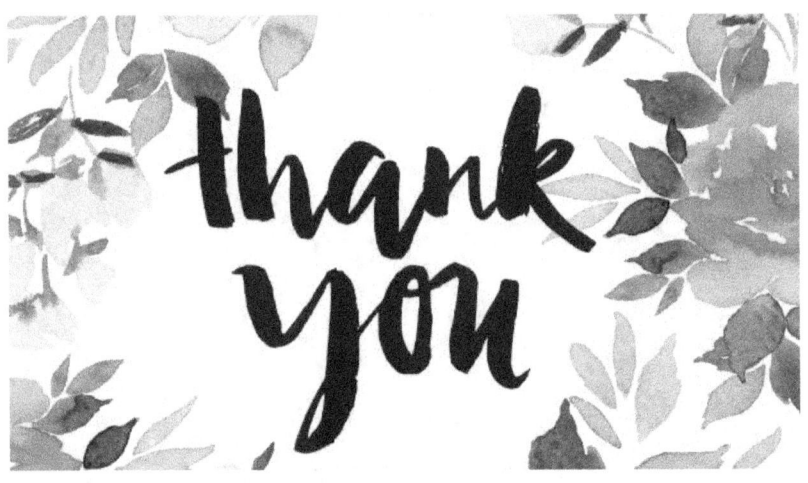

Disclaimer Notice:

Please note the information contained within this document is for educational and entertainment purposes only. Every attempt has been made to provide accurate, up to date and reliable, complete information. No warranties of any kind are expressed or implied. Readers acknowledge that the author is not engaging in the rendering of legal, financial, medical or professional advice.

By reading this document, the reader agrees that under no circumstances are we responsible for any losses, direct or indirect, which are incurred as a result of the use of information contained in this document, including, but not limited to, —errors, omissions, or inaccuracies.